ALL THINGS GIRL

Modern and Modest

TERESA TOMEO
MOLLY MILLER
MONICA COPS

The "All Things Girl" series is published by
Bezalel Books
Waterford, MI
www.BezalelBooks.com

The titles in the ALL THINGS GIRL series are:

Friends, Boys, and Getting Along

Mirror, Mirror on the Wall...What is Beauty After All?

Girls Rock!

Mind Your Manners

Modern and Modest

All Things Girl Journal

"ATG" Mother-Daughter events can be scheduled through www.RunwaytoReality.org or by visiting www.TeresaTomeo.com.

References to the Catechism of the Catholic Church are denoted: CCC

ISBN 978-0-9818854-5-2
Library of Congress Control Number 2008931737

Table of Contents

To Cheryl, Molly, and Monica~
thanks for your witness, your
amazing Christian sisterhood, and
for including me in on
All Things Girl –
an extremely rewarding
and important project.
Let's hear it
for the girls!
T.

To my daughter, Lucy.
Love, Mom
To my nieces: Janet,
Maren and Emma, Maria,
Leah, Lydia, and Nadia.
You are all so beautiful!
Love, Aunt Molly

*To my dear friend Molly, who
has taught me all about fashion
and with whom I have spent
countless hours working,
praying and laughing together; I
am truly blessed for your
friendship! Love, Monica*

High Class

All people begin life in their mother's womb. From the beginning of your creation, tiny as you were, you were a person. Being created a person, and not, let's say, a kitty or a dog, is special because God gave you a soul that will live forever. A person is a creature made up of a body and a soul. As a person, you are in a "higher class" because your soul is what gives you "the image and likeness of God." Your Creator, God the Father has stamped on your soul, dignity. What is dignity? It is your worth as a person.

Dignity has three characteristics:

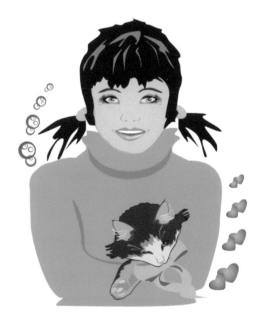

1) You have it no matter what circumstances you live in.

2) You have it no matter what you look like.

3) You have it, mo matter what changes you go through in your life.

Here are some examples

Jennifer lives in a neighborhood where the houses are very small and the people work hard but don't have much money. **Katie** lives in a mansion and takes expensive vacations every year. Which person has more dignity?

Jade is from Africa and has deep brown skin. **Julie** has red hair and freckles. **Laura** is chubby. **Maggie** is tall and skinny. Which girl has more dignity?

Opal is 95 years old and lives in a nursing home and has to be spoon fed. **Riley** was in a car accident and has a huge scar on her face. **Jessica** is a beautiful movie star. Which person has more dignity?

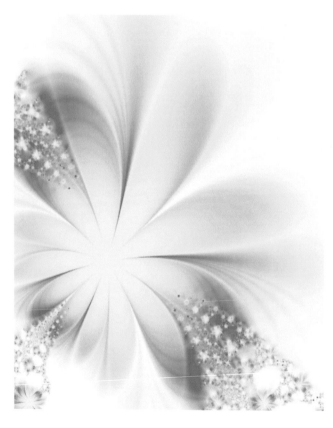

Hopefully you answered "neither" to all of the examples because all people are equal in dignity. You will go through good and bad times, happiness and sadness, success and failure in your life. Sometimes people think these things are what define you. This is a lie you must not believe. At this point you should be feeling pretty good about yourself. Just in case you need more, check it out, it gets better!

Princess

When you were a baby, your mom and dad brought you to church to be baptized. What does baptism do? It washes away original sin, makes you a child of God and fills your soul with grace. God is the King of the universe, and you are his daughter: that makes you a princess! *As a princess in the royal family of God, you have a value greater than a rare jewel* and He loves you soooooo much. This is what defines you as a person and nothing, including popularity, good grades, designer clothes or money, makes a difference in who you are in the sight of God your Father.

So you see, you are so much more than body parts. You are intelligent, creative and caring. You are not an object, but a person, and a female person at that! Sexuality is what makes you a girl, different from males. Only a woman can carry another living person within her body. *God also gave to women unique gifts such as a nurturing heart, a giving spirit, and a detail oriented mind.* These gifts are used for the good of those around you and for your own true happiness.

Lots of girls grow up trying to answer the soul searching question of *"Why am I here?"*

The answer is simple, *To know, love, and serve God in this life and to be happy with Him forever in Heaven in the next.* You get to *know, love and serve God from Jesus Christ, the Son of God, who teaches us through the Catholic Church.*

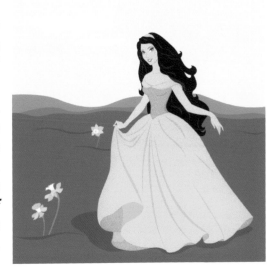

But how do you do all these? Let's go step by step:

1. How do you know God?

What would you do if you want to get to know a movie star? You try to read up all the information about him or her in magazines and books, you would watch interviews on TV., ask people around you what they know, etc. Well, you get to know God in a similar way: Reading the Bible, listening to your parents talk about God, listening in religion class seriously, praying and receiving the Sacraments.

2. How do you get to love a person?

Well, by spending time with them. To love God, you also need to spend time with Him in prayer, adoring and thanking Him for your blessings, and worshipping Him at Sunday Mass.

3. How do you serve God?

You serve God by serving other people. Serving God is doing daily chores cheerfully without complaining, or participating in service projects.

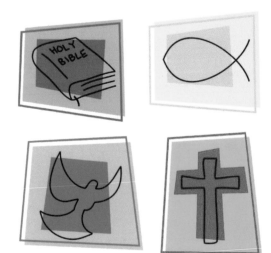

As you grow up, ask Our Lord in what special way He wants you to know, love and serve Him. This will be your vocation and will make you truly happy in your life.

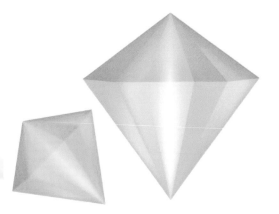

Ok, now you realize that you are a princess, a daughter of the King. The trick is to show you really believe this fact.

You have to live it!

What kind of things will show that you know that you are worth more than a rare jewel? Well, to begin with, the way you treat others is a real indicator that you realize you are a rare jewel. You get the fact that God loves you tremendously and so you are able to love others, as well.

Another way is to consider how you behave. These are things we talked about in Friends, Boys, and Getting Along. Remember the personality quiz? Now we will look at the fact that how you dress is a real show of your dignity as a daughter of the King, a princess. It's a way to express your personality and it tells a lot about a girl.

What is your fashion statement saying about you?
It should say "I am a daughter of the King!"

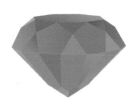

Fashion is important to a lot of girls your age but it is very important to realize that fashion is not always reasonable…

Here are a few interesting facts on how the fashion industry operates… What girls find attractive may not be comfortable or practical. But sadly girls will often put their own comfort aside to look fashionable. Think of spike heals and cute, tiny purses. If you look at the culture today you will be able to guess what is important in society. For example, in magazines and advertisements, you only see thin models, which tell you that being rail thin is beautiful and very important. But when a girl's bony shoulders are sticking out or her knees are knocking together, this isn't beauty, this is starvation.

Whatever is happening in the country is reflected in fashions. When there is war you will see styles that feature fatigues, somber colors and military type jackets. And don't forget that the industry recycles styles that have been popular before. Most of the time you can see things that were popular thirty years ago, resurface. Take, for example, argyle vests and sweaters: they were all the rage in the 1980's and in the mid 2000's they are popular again. There's a catch though. There is always something different the second time around so that it's not quite the same. For instance, the colors may be different or the fabric has changed.

It's a fact: The fashion industry is not interested in making girls feel good about themselves.

What this industry is interested in is your money! Don't be fooled. It is a multi-million-dollar business and it changes what it says is "fashionable" every year just so it can make money. But don't despair…You can have an impact on this giant industry by your buying patterns. If you and your friends support brand names and stores that show girls and guys wearing very skimpy clothing, these companies will continue to produce clothing that belittles the dignity of the person. On the other hand, if you and your friends choose name brands and stores that hold up your dignity by giving you modern and stylish options that cover intimate parts of the body, you can give the message that they should continue to make these clothing options available by spending your dollars at their stores and their brands.

Girls,
you always have power!

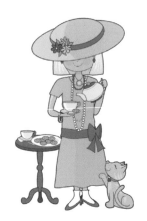

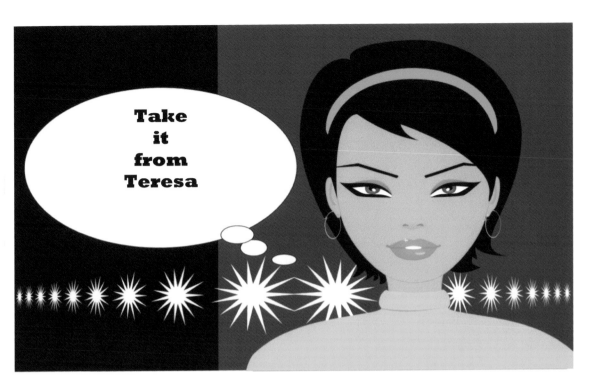

Take it from Teresa

You are not an item on display to be gawked at, or stared at, or judged for your appearance. You are a precious daughter of the King! Take it from me girls; in this media-saturated culture we live in, that statement sometimes can be a tough one to remember and to live up to. Have you ever heard the phrase "objectification of women" or how about just the word "objectification?" The phrase, and the word, means to be treated as an object, or a thing, that is used by someone. Think how sad that sounds: "used" by someone. Do you want to be "used?" Do you want to "use" others? Of course not! But, unfortunately because of all the pressure in today's culture which stresses appearance over soul and substance, more and more young women (all of whom are created in the image and likeness of God) are allowing themselves to be used. This will always make them feel less than dignified. Women are not meant to be valued only in regards to how they dress or how they act around boys, instead of who they are as a person. Women are meant to be valued for being created in the image and likeness of God! You, young lady, are a daughter of the King and are growing into a woman whose value comes directly from that status as princess.

The late Pope John Paul II was very concerned about the treatment of women in the culture. He addressed this topic in several ground breaking letters and Church documents, including his 1988 letter "*On the Dignity and Vocation of Women*" and another letter written in 1995 entitled "*Papal Letter to Women.*" John Paul II expressed a deep desire to right many of the wrongs in society which objectified women, including what he called a certain type of conditioning or way of thinking and looking at women which has occurred for centuries.

"This has prevented women from truly being themselves, and it has resulted in a spiritual impoverishment of humanity..."

Our late Holy Father was truly disturbed by a trend which showed a great disrespect for women and did not reflect how Jesus viewed His precious daughters.

"When it comes to setting women free from every kind of exploitation and domination, the Gospel contains an ever relevant message which goes back to the attitude of Jesus Christ himself. Transcending the established norms of his own culture, Jesus treated women with openness, respect, acceptance and tenderness. In this way he honored the dignity which women have always possessed according to God's plan and in his love."

You might be familiar with the many Bible passages where our Lord encounters women along His journey and treats them as the late Pope explained, with "openness, respect, acceptance, and tenderness." In Chapter 4 of St. John's Gospel, Jesus meets the Samaritan woman at the well. He restores her dignity by telling her about the "living water" only He can give. St. Martha and St. Mary or, the 'Women of Bethany' as they are also known, became a key part of His ministry,

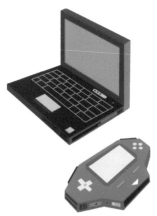

along with St. Mary Magdalene. Did you know that St. Mary Magdalene was the first to see our risen Lord on the very first Easter Sunday? Maybe this doesn't sound so impressive to you because you are blessed to live during a time where women and girls have all kinds of different opportunities. But in Jesus' day it certainly wasn't the case. As a matter of fact women were considered property and if you needed a witness in a court of law only the testimony of men was allowed! That's why Jesus thought it was so important for EVERYONE to understand that God created women with great dignity and value. We don't want our world going back to the time before Jesus when women were often objects and not daughters of the King.

The Bible and the Catholic Church uphold our dignity and also teach us that our bodies are temples of the Holy Spirit. As you have been learning in this book and the entire *All Things Girls* series, moderation (being modern and modest) is key when it comes to dressing nicely and taking care of yourself, both inside and out. We do all things to glorify God and to be holy in His sight. Your outside should reflect your inside. Your clothing should reflect that you know what it means to be a daughter of the King.

In February of 2007 a professional group of psychologists released an eye-opening study about this problem of objectification of girls. These experts found that girls who are portrayed in a certain less lady-like way, in TV commercials and programs, magazine ads and articles, as well as music videos and other media outlets, end up feeling used or "objectified." There's that word again: object. Are you an object or a person? Don't let yourself become an object and if you are feeling like an object, talk to your mom or dad. Help yourself feel right again. These feelings of "objectification," the report found, can lead to many problems including to self-esteem issues, eating disorders, and depression.

Other studies have found that the media, in general, can make girls feel pretty bad about themselves because they might feel they don't matter much if they don't look like one of the favorite pop stars on television or the runway models.

And no wonder. Every time you turn around you are bombarded with pictures and images that dwell on the outside of a person and not the inside of a person, which is what really counts. But the fine line here is to remember that we still ought to take care to be clean and mindful of our appearance. It just shouldn't be where we put our emphasis when understanding "true beauty."

Get a load of this...one out of every four TV commercials contains a message about appearance and 80% of women questioned, not too long ago, by *People Magazine* said media images make them feel insecure. Imagine letting media make you feel insecure! I'm telling you, girlfriend, don't let that happen. Don't let air-brushed, computer-enhanced images be your "ideal" person. Think about it, these aren't what real people even look like on their best day!

And did you know that even music videos featuring thin women lead to an increase in body dissatisfaction; so much so that one out of every three women in this country is on a diet at any given time. No wonder the folks who sell diet programs and products make up 35 billion dollars in sales every year! That "b" looks like that on purpose. We're talking billions, that's a whole lot of hard earned money being spent because the media has convinced us we aren't all we should be in the looks department.

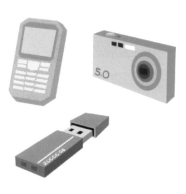

This comes as no surprise to yours truly. I developed an eating disorder because I wanted to look like my favorite TV actress and I let my classmates in grade school convince me that I wasn't good enough. My destructive eating habits put me in the hospital. Unfortunately, because not only the messages but the media outlets themselves have multiplied greatly since I was a teen, your challenge to remain modern but modest is a lot harder. And too many young girls have bought into the lies with 81% of ten year olds in America admitting they are afraid of being fat. I don't recommend being afraid of anything but of being fat? Yikes. If anything we should be afraid of not remembering how awesome it is to be a daughter of the King!

Anyhow, this can be a vicious cycle and very confusing for you. You may be feeling great pressure to dress in a less than modest way to get more attention or feel more important. But eventually that attention will make you feel more like a 'thing' than a person, because others are being attracted to you for the wrong reasons and just like that report from the mental health experts suggests, you might start feeling pretty bad about yourself. Or you might be comparing yourself to certain images on screen or in print and feeling insecure or unhappy.

What's a Godly girl like you to do? Well we know we should turn away from the media and turn to Jesus and the Church for our real identity, so here are a few suggestions to help you as you do your best to be modern and modest:

- Talk to your parents about doing a "media reality check" in your home. Sit down and take a look at just how much time you are spending on the computer or watching TV. The experts say no more than two hours of TV a day for teens and tweens.
- Help your family form a "family media plan" which involves keeping the computer and TV in the family room, and finding good family friendly movies, programs, and games.
- Remember the commandment to honor your Mother and Father and cooperate with your parents when it comes to media restrictions.

◉ Look toward heaven and not Hollywood and find your role models in the Communion of Saints, especially our Blessed Mother.

As John Paul II tells us, over the years there have been many great examples of women who were both modern and modest in their own way in their own time making a major mark on the world. He said...

"In a particular way I think of St. Catherine of Siena and of St. Teresa of Avila, whom Pope Paul VI of happy memory granted the title of doctors of the church. And how can we overlook the many women, inspired by faith, who were responsible for initiatives of extraordinary social importance, especially in serving the poorest of the poor?"

St. Catherine of Siena reminds us "when we are who we are called to be, we will sent the world ablaze."

So come on, as that old saying goes, let's put our best foot forward for Christ!

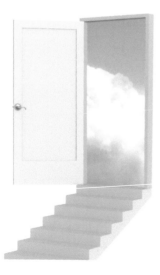

Always remember:
You are intended for an eternal life with God!

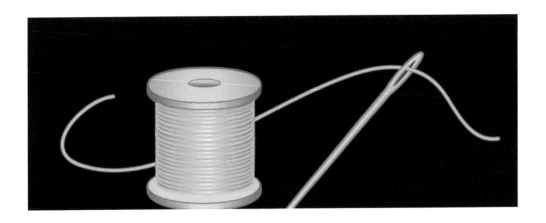

Fashion and Fabrics 101

Girls today don't always get the opportunity to learn sewing. This is a pity because sewing is the essence of fashion. All designers know how to sew and make patterns. If you have a great idea for a dress or coat, just drawing a picture won't cut it! You have to know how to put garments together, how to choose the right fabric, how fabrics feel and look and how to make the garment fit a real human body.

Let's start from scratch. This book will give you a very basic introduction to styles and fabrics so that you can begin to understand fashion. You will then be able to make better choices in the market place using this knowledge. You can impress your friends with your new expertise on fashion!

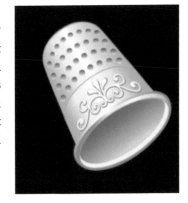

Read through the next few pages very carefully and be ready to take the fashion quiz that follows! Don't be surprised if you ask your mom or dad to hook you up with some sewing lessons at the local fabric and craft store. It would be a great new sort of birthday or Christmas present to ask for instead of the same 'ol, same 'ol. You'll have fun and learn a whole new skill.

Fabrics

Natural Fabrics

- ➤ Cotton - Comes from the cotton plant. It is cool, comfortable, and easy to clean. Examples include t-shirt material and denim. It wrinkles and shrinks easily.
- ➤ Linen - Made from the flax plant. It is cool, comfortable and can be hand washed or dry-cleaned. Jackets and skirts are made from linen as a spring fabric. It is known for wrinkling.
- ➤ Wool - Comes form animals such as sheep, goats and llamas. It is a warm fiber and is made into sweaters, jackets, skirts and pants. It can be hand washed or dry-cleaned depending on the garment. Some people find it to feel itchy on their skin. It should be stored with lavender, moth balls or in a cedar closet to keep moths from eating holes in garments made of wool.
- ➤ Silk - Made by silk worms. It is the strongest fiber. Blouses, scarves, dresses, jackets, skirts and pants can be made from it. It can be quite expensive. Some silk can be hand washed but most garments should be dry cleaned.

Synthetic Fabrics

- ➤ Spandex - A very stretchy manmade fiber that is woven with other fibers to make garments that are comfortable and gives "move-ability" to them.
- ➤ Rayon - A soft manmade fiber that is used for skirts, blouses and dresses. It is comfortable but wrinkles easily. It should be dry-cleaned. It is known to shrink when washed, even by hand.
- ➤ Polyester - Is a very versatile manmade fiber, which can be woven with any fiber to make the garment more comfortable and easier to launder.

Modesty protects the intimate center of the person. It means refusing to unveil what should remain hidden.
CCC#2521

Read the definitions and see how much you can remember for the fashion challenge on the next page.

Skirts

1. A line-fitted at the waist and hips with a flare at the bottom
2. Pencil-fitted at the waist and hips and narrows at the knees
3. Gored-fitted at the waist and hips with fullness past the knees
4. Straight-fitted at the waist and hips
5. Peasant-fitted at the waist with soft, flowing bottom

Pants

6. Capri - Short pants cut above the ankle.
7. Straight Leg - A cut of pants that fall straight from the hip.
8. Pencil Leg - A fitted leg that narrows at the ankle.
9. Flared Leg - The pant leg fits in the hips and thighs and widens at the ankle.
10. Leggings - Form fitting leg coverings made of stretch fabric and hug the leg.

Tops

Types of Sleeves:

11. Dolman - A long sleeve that is very wide at the top and narrow at the wrist.
12. Set in - A sleeve, long or short that is sewn into the armhole of the top.
13. Raglan - A sleeve that extends from the neckline and in not "set in."
14. Cap - A very short sleeve not going past the armpit.

Types of Collars:

15. Notched - The type of collar seen on suit jackets, resembling a pair or wings with a triangle cut out of it.
16. Shawl - A rounded collar on a V-neckline.
17. Mandarin - A small standup collar and open in the front.

Types of Necklines:

18. Jewel neckline - Also called a T-shirt neckline is a circular shape around the neck.
19. Scoop neckline - A U shaped neckline.
20. Boat neckline - A neckline which is two lines going across the collar bone.
21. V necklines - Two lines starting at shoulder and meeting on the chest and shaped like a V.
22. Square necklines – Are shaped like a square around the neck.

Ready for the fashion challenge? Fill in the numbers from the previous explanations. Hint: some have two answers. You'll find the answers on page 25.

Row 1: ___ ___ ___ ___ ___ ___

Row 2: ___ ___ ___ ___ ___ ___

Row 3: ___ ___ ___ ___ ___ ___

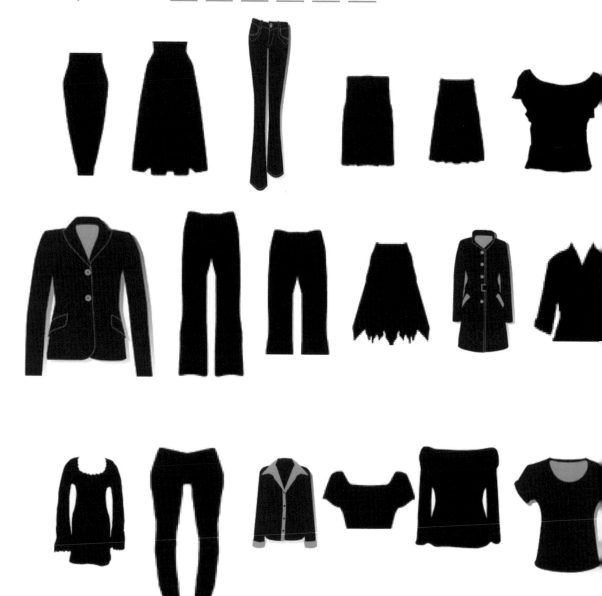

Refusing to Unveil...

Now that you have a basic idea of styles and fabrics in fashion, let's get down to some issues that impact your choices in fashion. Let's face it, our culture emphasizes outward beauty. While we all appreciate a pretty face, this of course is not the value of the person. This topic is discussed in *Mirror, Mirror on the Wall, What is Beauty After All?* However, it is perfectly reasonable to want to look your best and wear things that are in style. With the help and influence of your mother and dad, you certainly can have some choices. With these choices though, there is responsibility, even in fashion.

You know, modesty has gotten a bad "rap" lately. It brings to mind images of styles that a lot of girls don't like. But it is important to separate what the culture says you should wear and what you really should wear. The Catechism of the Catholic Church gives a beautiful definition of modesty, which is, "refusing to unveil which should remain hidden." Each girl has intimate parts that make her a girl, a woman. The breasts, the midriff, the bottom are the parts of your body that you have a right and a responsibility to keep private. This is modesty. It protects you from others viewing you as an object.

With this in mind, here's some ways that you can be modest but modern! First of all, always remember, you are a princess, a member of the royal of God. This is a gift and a privilege. When you are choosing, with your mother's help and approval, your clothing, remember to pay attention to what others will see as the focal point!

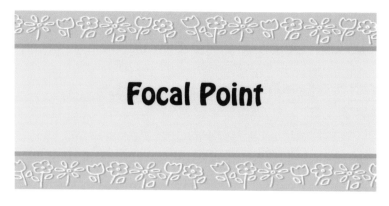

Focal Point

Focal point is simply, where the focus is. It is the first place the eye is attracted. It is said that the eyes are the windows to the soul, and the soul is what animates the body. This is where you want others' attention to be when they are looking at you. Have you ever been talking to someone and they look past you or over your shoulder? How does that feel? Like you're being ignored, or that what you are saying doesn't mean anything? Yah, not so good.

The best way to keep attention on the face is to keep attention OFF the private parts of your body. This would mean the bust line, midriff, and bottom. By "refusing to unveil which must remain hidden," you are allowing people to notice you, not your body parts. Other practical ways to keep attention on your face are:

- Wear a cute hairstyle.
- Wear accessories such as necklaces or earrings, if your mom thinks this is appropriate for you.
- SMILE!

Purity requires modesty, an integral part of temperance. Modesty protects the intimate center of the person. It means refusing to unveil what should remain hidden.
CCC# 2521

Layering

When shopping for tops, make sure they are long enough in the body to cover your midriff and your back when you bend over. Sometimes it's not that the tops aren't long enough, but your pants are cut too low. If your lower back and "bottom" show, your pants are *way* too low. There are many options now so choose jeans or pants that will keep your backside "under wraps." It's very distracting for others, boys, men, and other women when at Church, in the library or at school, to have to look at the girl in front of them with half her bottom showing because her pants are just too low. You can also choose to layer your garments to insure "skin coverage." There are many cute camis out there to purchase to make sure you don't show anything that should remain hidden. A great layering piece is the men's sleeveless white undershirts. They are long, they fit close to the body, they are lightweight and they can be turned backward to cover in the front.

WARNING: Under no circumstances are undergarments to be worn alone!!!

Undergarments

While on the subject of layering, undergarments are part of this discussion. Recently, a popular celeb was making it known that she did not wear panties. So, rule number one, always wear underpants!!! Seems like a no-brainer, but judging from Hollywood and the like, people missed that lesson!

At some point you will need to wear a bra for the sake of modesty. Following is a chart to help you and mom know how to pick the right size and style for you. Many stores will help fit you if you ask. Mom, you need to do this too for yourself. Wearing the correct size and style of bra for you will be comfortable and will even make you look better!

How to Fit a Bra

1. Measure all the way around just above your breasts for band size: i.e., 36 inches equals a size-36 bra.
2. For cup size, measure across the fullest part of your breasts. Then subtract the band size from that number.
3. Consult the chart to find your cup size.

AA	½"
A	1"
B	2"
C	3"
D	4"
DD or E	5"
F	6"
G	7"

Types of Bras

❖ Sports- fits close to the body and keeps the breasts flat
❖ Soft Cups-fits according to size with a hook back and adjustable straps
❖ Molded Cups-fits according to size with a hook back and adjustable straps and slightly padded cups.

When choosing a bra with mom's help, purchase the type that is comfortable. Here are a few tips on finding the correct fit for you.

-   The back of the bra should lay flat and straight. If it rides up, it is too small around.
-   If the cups wrinkle, they are too big and you should go down a cup size.
-   If you have cleavage showing, the cup size is too small: go up one size.
-   If your breasts are showing underneath, the straps are "hiked up" too far and need to be let down.

Fashion challenge answers for the quiz on page 19.
So? How'd you do?

Row 1:   2, 3, 9, 4, 1, 14&19
Row 2:   12 & 16, 7, 6, 5, 12 &17, 11 &21
Row 3:   13 & 19, 10 & 8, 15, 22, 20, 14 &18

When choosing panties...

100% cotton is the best. Remember what you learned about the natural fibers above, cotton is comfortable and it breathes. This can prevent infections and keep you cool and comfy. Whatever style you and mom decide on, just remember it is underwear and should remain under your clothing. This is a general rule of thumb that applies to any underwear, including bra straps. It is inappropriate for bra straps, colored or plain, to show, even though it is popular to have several straps showing from bras, camis, and tanks.

Remember, you are a member of the royal family of God and knowing this, you want to look the part. If a girl has her bra straps showing, others become curious. Protect yourself and others from undue curiosity and keep things covered!

Modesty inspires a way of life which makes it possible to resist the allurements of fashion and the pressures of prevailing ideologies.
CCC#2523

Fashion Personality Quiz

Directions: Answer the questions with your initial reaction. Add up letters at the end.

1. A casual outfit for myself would be:

a) Athletic pants, a tee shirt or sweatshirt
b) Jeans, khakis, button down shirt or polo
c) Pants with ruffled shirt and lace cami underneath
d) Pants or jeans, knit top with a chunky necklace, bracelet and large earrings
e) Jeans and a knobby cotton pull over shirt

2. Accessories I would choose are:

a) I seldom wear accessories
b) Scarves, pins or necklace sets
c) Pearls, cameos, lace shawls and collars
d) Bold chunky necklaces, big earrings, bright colored scarves and fur collars
e) Shell or macramé necklaces, leather bracelets

3. An ensemble I would wear to a wedding is:

a) A knit skirt or pant set
b) A tailored suit or dress
c) A floral dress
d) A dressy suit with rhinestones
e) A broomstick skirt with a gauzy top

4. My favorite type of shoes are:

a) Tennis shoes or slides
b) Loafers or traditional pump
c) Ballet slipper or a pump with a bow on the toe
d) The hottest new thing out there
e) Birkenstocks

5. My favorite fabric pattern would be:

   a) Solids or stripes
   b) Solids, plaids, herring bone or tweed
   c) Flora or lace
   d) Animal print, geometric
   e) No real patterns, but soft natural textures

6. My favorite top would be:

   a) Tee shirt or sweatshirt
   b) Button down blouse or polo
   c) Ruffled blouse
   d) Black knit with fur trim at the neck and sleeves
   e) Denim shirt

So? What did you find out about yourself?

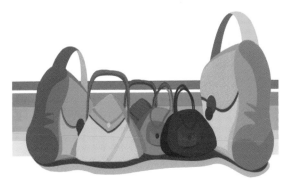

Mostly A's: You are a sporty gal! You are most comfortable in athletic wear and tennis shoes. You don't like to dress up or wear accessories. Your main goal is comfort.

Mostly B's: You are a classic young woman. You love the styles that change very little. Button down shirts, blazers and basic skirts in timeless black, navy and red are your favorites. You dress these pieces up or down for the occasion.

Mostly C's: You are a romantic at heart. You love to look and feel feminine. You choose lace and florals and feel pretty in them. Long, flowing skirts are a favorite.

Mostly D's: You have a dramatic flair! You love attention and you wear things others are afraid of. You love being on the cutting edge of fashion. Your wardrobe is full of basic black, bold accessories and wild prints.

Mostly E's: You love a natural look and feel. You are happy with natural fibers, cotton, linen and wool. Sometimes your style resembles a hippie or hobo look. You take your cue from nature.

It's Gotta Fit

There's a lot to be said about how a garment fits. A few little fashion rules will help you. First of all, things worn too big appear to be sloppy and add weight to the body. Things that are tight, say across the bust line, will become your focal point. Girls, you don't want that!

The right fit allows you to move, bend, raise your arms and not be worried about skin showing. It's too tight if:

❖ The buttons on your blouse gap open.
❖ Your t-shirt pulls and wrinkles across the bust line.
❖ You can't move comfortably.
❖ The pleats on your pants don't lay flat.
❖ Your tummy pooches over your pants. (AKA muffin top.)

The Bottom Line

Girls, you are beautiful and so special. Don't blindly follow the trend if it's not covering what should remain hidden. There are great options that are cool, hip, and stylish. You don't have to settle. Just in case you are a black and white kinda gal, here are a few guidelines for modesty.

❖ Whatever neckline you choose, be sure that you don't show cleavage. Bend over and look in the mirror to make sure you can't see all the way to China!
❖ Make sure the fabric of the garment skims, not hugs the body.
❖ All undergarments should be covered including bra straps.
❖ If you can't comfortably bend down to pick up your pencil, it's too short, whether it's shorts or skirts.
❖ If you bend over and your back shows, your top is too short or your pants are too low.
❖ Fabrics should not be sheer.

Swim Suits

With the return recently of the string bikini, many girls are at the beach almost naked! Come on, think about this! Practically naked! Can you even imagine that this is okay with your Father in heaven? Remember the big fashion question you answered earlier?

What is your fashion statement saying about you?
It should say "I am a daughter of the King!"

This is something very serious to remember when you and your mom go shopping for a bathing suit...

Every girl, every woman is created with a very special gift. This gift is the ability to carry a life within their bodies! Our Lady is called the Ark of the Covenant because she carried Jesus in her womb. She is your role model in that way and in the ways in which you want to live as a daughter of the King.

Because of this priceless gift, the womb, the midriff should be protected and hidden. It is to be respected. A way to do that is to cover and veil this area. It is sacred. Imagine that! What a gift God has given you. And what a responsibility you have to protect that gift. This is why it's good to avoid two-piece swimsuits. Maybe this seems silly or maybe you "get it" but either way, you should consider this with mom when you get your next suit.

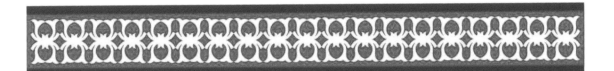

Daddy's Little Girl

Just as you are God the Father's little girl, you are your earthly father's daughter as well. Dads are super important to girls growing up. Good fathers teach their daughters how to be respected by boys. He does this by his example. Watch how he treats your mother and his own mother. He protects you and watches out for your best interest. He wants the best for you. He gives you an image of your Heavenly Father. Because of this, it's dad's job to make sure you dress as a daughter of the King. Dads know what it's like to be a young man. They know how boys think and feel. If your dad ever asks you to change your clothes or doesn't want you to wear something, listen to him. He is protecting you. It's a pain to change when you are ready to go someplace, but do it without arguing and without a fuss. It won't take long and you will know that your dad loves you and is always looking out for your best interests. Your dad is a gift from God.

Sadly, some girls don't have their dads around because of either divorce or death. But no girl should ever despair! Girls always have a Dad in God. Look to Him and let Him comfort and protect you. Your Heavenly Father will always be there for you! What is super-cool about your Father in heaven is that He made a special place in your heart for His indwelling. That means that no matter where you go, or what you do, God is with you. It is also how He talks to you. This is a beautiful relationship you will continue to develop your whole life so just because you don't have an earthly father in your life doesn't mean you don't have a Dad! Go ahead, talk to your Heavenly Father today, He's waiting to hear from you!

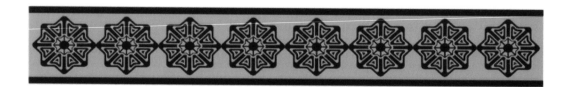

Look to Mom

Just as Dad is important in the whole fashion scheme of things, so is Mom. She is your first example of fashion, like it or not. If your mom isn't your idea of a fashion icon, here's some food for thought...

Honor your father and mother, that you may have a long life in the land which the Lord, your God, is giving you.
Exodus 20:12

After having babies, women's bodies change. Many women gain a few pounds and the fashions that look good on a teenager won't look good on a mature woman. Along those same lines, what is appropriate for a young woman to wear is not so for mom. Moms know better! You can probably imagine all sorts of things you wear and your mom wouldn't or couldn't. And aren't you glad, really, if you think about it?!

That's not to say mom shouldn't take care of her appearance and wear stylish clothing. It's just a fact that mom shouldn't look like a teenybopper.

Another consideration is that your mom may have a different fashion personality than you. Have her take the test, too, and see what you have in common and what is different. You are both unique with your own ideas and preferences, your own likes and dislikes. These are to be respected and embraced. If you are choosing clothing that doesn't veil that which should remain hidden, then mom and you may disagree on styles. With this in mind, mom has the last word on your choices. These are all things to discuss BEFORE you go shopping together. Fighting with your mom at the store is a big no-no. It isn't what a daughter of the King does. Like it or not, but hopefully you like it, God gave you the mother you have and the Bible says that you are supposed to honor her and your father. That's a commandment so, either way, there's no getting out of it!

THE WEDDING VEIL

You know, history can be very interesting if you just give it a chance. Did you ever wonder why brides wear veils? There are many traditions that have made their way through history. The ancient Greeks and Romans were superstitious and believed that the veil covering the bride protected her from evil spirits. In the Middle Ages many parents arranged marriages for their children. This was very common with kings so that they could unite kingdoms and make their territory larger. In that case, the bride was veiled until after the vows, in the case that the bride was homely and the groom wanted to change his mind. Talk about degrading women! It didn't seem to matter what the bride thought of her groom. In Jewish tradition, the bride wears a veil to symbolize the fact that physical beauty fades and it is what's inside that counts. Now that shows understanding of the beauty and dignity of a person! That is what the Church is all about, too! Cool, isn't it?

The soul and the modesty of the bride are what is really important. Later in history, veiling became a symbol of purity and modesty. Today there are many styles of veils brides wear, but most of the tradition symbolizing purity and modesty has all but disappeared and the veil is only part of the décor for the wedding costume. If you marry one day, if that is the vocation to which God calls you, you may want to consider veiling your face to recall the beautiful tradition symbolizing the virtue of the bride.

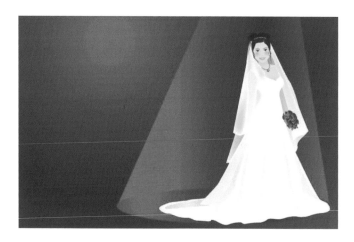

Dress for the Occasion

In days gone by, women wore different types of clothing for different occasions. Today, around our country, it seems anything goes. What you wear to a picnic also passes for going out to eat, to a party, and even to Mass. This is very sad that society has gotten so casual and relaxed. People have forgotten how fun it is to be dressed up and to have special clothes for special occasions. God says we are "put aside" for Him and we ought to have certain things "put aside" to mark different times, like a party or Mass.

When we don't mark things like Church attendance as any different than, let's say, shopping at the mall, it belittles the dignity of the person. Why? Because how a person dresses shows how she feels about herself. Here are a couple fashion rules of thumb:

- *Pajamas, boxers and the like are only for the home or a sleepover.*
- *Shorts, t-shirts, capris, are fine for casual outings such as a picnic or barbeque.*
- *Sweats and athletic wear are for the gym, and sporting events.*

When attending a wedding, a dinner or Mass, a skirt or dress is really the best way to go. If a person dresses up to meet say, the President of the United States of America, so, too, we should dress up for our God, our King and our Savior. There are always exceptions to the rule, but the norm is to kick it up a notch for Mass.

*H*ere are some things to avoid wearing to Mass:

- Strappy tank tops, halters and camisoles (These should be avoided anywhere you go!)
- Shorts
- Jeans with holes
- Low cut jeans and tops
- Mini skirts and tight pants

*I*nstead try:

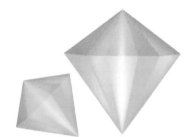

- Cute blazers and sweater sets
- Skirts and dresses
- Pants and blouses

*S*tart a trend and be the one to bring a little formality back into fashion. You'll see, its fun to dress up for different occasions.

Modesty is decency.
It inspires one's choice of clothing.
CCC#2522

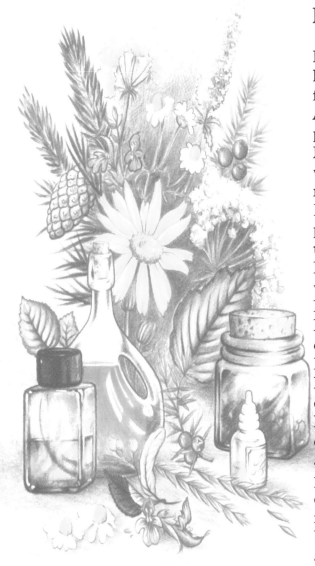

PERFUME: HUNGARY WATER

Did you know that people have been wearing perfume for many, many centuries? Actually, the art of making perfume began in ancient Mesopotamia and Egypt, but was developed and further refined by the Romans and the Persians. The first modern perfume was made in 1370, at the request of Queen Elizabeth of Hungary, and it was known throughout Europe as "Hungary Water". In the 16th Century, Catherine of Medici, who was married to King Henry II, from France, hired Rene Le Florentin to create personal perfumes for her. His laboratory was connected with her apartments by a secret passageway, so that no one could steal Le Florentin's formulas. France quickly became the center of perfume and cosmetic manufacture of the whole Europe, and it remains today as such! During this time, perfumes were used only by royalty and the wealthy to mask body odors. By the 18th century, aromatic plants were grown in France with the special purpose of creating perfumes.

PERFUME FACTS:

- Perfumes are a mixture of essential oils, aroma compounds and solvents used to give the human body a pleasant odor.
- Originally perfume was worn to hide unpleasant body odors; nowadays, perfume is used also to make a personal statement and even to please the person that wears it!
- Perfume is made up of animal or plant-based aromatic compounds such as botanical oils, animal musk's oils or nowadays synthetic scents that come from different chemicals.
- The compound is dissolved in a mixture of alcohol and water. Depending on how much water is used to dissolve the aromatic compound, the blend becomes a perfume or cologne.
- True perfume contains the least amount of water and alcohol. But true perfumes are rarely sold, because they are very expensive to make.
- You may have seen the words "Eau du parfum" in some perfume bottles; these words mean that this particular perfume contains more water and alcohol than a true perfume. "Eau du parfums" are the perfumes that most people wear and are more familiar with.
- "Eau du Cologne" is a more lightly scented perfume that can be applied more liberally after a bath or shower.
- Another type of perfume is perfume oil. The compound is mixed with oil instead of alcohol and water. People with dry skin prefer these kind of perfumes, since the alcohol based perfumes have a tendency to dry the skin more. These kinds of perfumes can be formulated into "solid" perfumes that can be rubbed on the skin.

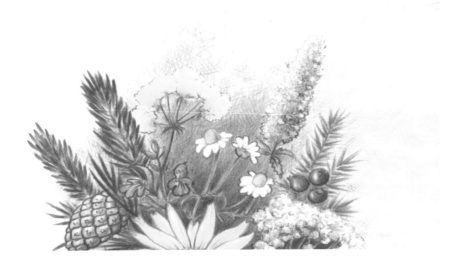

TYPES OF FRAGRANCES:

Read the descriptions below for the different types of fragrances. Which one is you?

- ○ Floral: It's created mainly from flowers, such as orange blossoms, roses, gardenias, jasmines and carnations. Sometimes the flower scents are mixed together. Their scent is very sweet, good for sweet, romantic women.
- ○ Oriental: These luxurious fragrances are created from a mix of spices, amber, balsams and resins. These are good for women who are daring and like to stand out of the crowd.
- ○ Citrus or Fruity: These are made from citrus fruit such as tangerine, lime, lemon and mandarin; they project a tangy aroma. These fragrances are good for women who like to be natural and feel fresh and don't want to wear an overpowering perfume.
- ○ Green: These are a blend of pine, leaves, juniper and herbs; their scent is sporty, good for women who love action and the outdoors!

Perfume How to's

You don't want to be like the girl on the school bus who had so much perfume on that everybody had to open the windows to get some air to breathe! The poor bus driver couldn't even drive straight! This is why it is important for you to learn basic tips on how to apply perfume, as well as making it last.

1. Apply your perfume before you put on any clothing or jewelry. Some perfumes will leave permanent stains on your clothing and jewelry.
2. Apply a small amount of perfume to your body pulse points: wrists, behind your ear lobes, throat, in the bend of your elbows and between your breasts. Sometimes, its just enough to spray your finger and rub it gently in each of the pulse points.
3. After you apply perfume to your wrists, don't rub them together; this breaks down the scent!
4. You may apply a small amount of perfume to your hair if it's freshly washed. If not, your hair's natural oils will change the perfume scent and you may end up with a bad fragrance in your hair! To apply perfume to your hair, you may want to spray your hands with perfume and then disperse it through your hair, or you may spray it directly on your hair at a distance of at least 8 inches.
5. Place your perfume in cool place to make the original scent last longer.

DISCUSS WITH YOUR MOM WHEN IT IS APPROPRIATE FOR YOU TO START WEARING PERFUME. HAVE FUN PICKING A FRAGRANCE THAT EXPRESSES YOUR PERSONALITY!

DO YOU KNOW WHAT PURITY REALLY IS?

Before you read the definition and explanation of this virtue, take the quiz. Remember: Be honest with yourself!

1) You're at school after gym class. All the girls are changing and getting dressed. You:

A) Mind your own business and get dressed as fast as you can.
B) You look around curiously at the other girls and compare yourself to them.
C) You notice other girls and wish you had their bodies instead of your own.

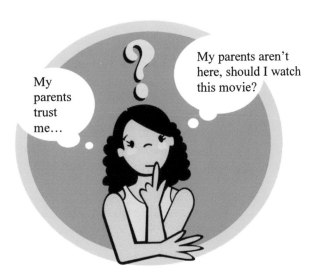

2) You're listening to music with your friends. A song comes on that uses nasty words. You:

A) Suggest listening to another song.
B) Realize the words are bad but are too embarrassed to say anything to your friends so you just keep quiet.
C) Sing along to the nasty song.

3) You are at a friend's for a sleepover with a couple other friends. They want to watch a movie rated PG13 and one that you know your parents would not let you watch. You:

A) Suggest other movies until another is chosen.
B) Go along with the girls and close your eyes at the bad scenes.
C) Ignore what you know your parents would think and go along with the girls.

4) Your sister is on the phone with the door shut. You are curious so you:

A) Ask her about it later when she is off the phone.
B) Listen at the door to see what you can hear.
C) Pick up the other extension and listen quietly.

5) Your favorite pen is missing. You:

A) Figure you lost it or left it at home.
B) Assume the boy sitting next to you stole it but keep it to yourself.
C) Accuse the boy sitting next to you of stealing your pen and tell everyone you know that he's a thief.

6) You get an unsigned note that says, "Nobody likes you." Later you find out one of your "friends" wrote it. You:

A) Ask your friend why she did that and say a prayer for her, knowing something must be wrong.
B) Start imagining what you can do to get her back.
C) You write a list all her faults and pass it around the entire grade getting signatures. After you get everyone to sign the list you tape it to your friend's locker, just to get her back.

7) One of your friends is talking with a teacher. You just have to know what the scoop is so you:

A) Go about your business and ask your friend later what the deal was.
B) Start imagining what they are talking about.
C) Walk by and drop your books so you can eavesdrop.

Key:
All A's: You have a pure heart. You guard your senses well by being careful what you look at and hear. Keep doing what you're doing.

All B's or a combination of A's and B's. You know what is good and pure, but you are not always willing to do the right thing, especially when friends are around. Practice following your conscience and pray for help from your guardian angel, or St. Maria Goretti and you will have a truly pure heart.

All C's or combination of B's and C's. Your heart is experiencing some pollution. You better clean it up by taking more care of what you look at, listen to, and think about. If you don't, your heart will become so dirty, it will be extremely difficult to get rid of all the pollutants. Ask your guardian angel and St. Maria Goretti to help you.

Virtues to Live by...

What is a virtue? Very simply, a virtue is a good habit that inclines you to do whatever is good. Virtuous behavior helps you live a good, happy life. But there is more to virtues than that. A single good action does not constitute a virtue. For instance, a person wouldn't be considered to have the virtue of generosity if she shared her candy with her friends only once. In order to become a virtue, a good habit has to be repeated on a regular basis.

Purity

The ultimate goal of every person is to get to Heaven. How do you get there? Purity of the heart is the way. How do you know this? Jesus says, "Blessed are the pure of heart for they shall see God."

So what does purity mean? Well, there's pure oxygen, pure water, pure chocolate and pure gold. That means they are free from foreign elements, impurities or pollutants. A pure heart is one that is clean, free of pollution. In order to keep a pure heart, think of the things that pollute the heart. There are certain movies, TV shows, books, advertisements, and magazines that can dirty the heart.

For example, immodestly dressed people, bad language, and impure relationships between men and women can give you ideas that are wrong and do affect you. These things leave a strong impression and if you are exposed to them, your heart can become impure.

Think about it...would you eat garbage out of a dumpster? Obviously, not. In the same way, don't put garbage into your mind so that it pollutes your heart.

You have the power to stay away from things that will make your heart and mind impure!

A pure heart also includes your thoughts, intentions, curiosity ,and judgment of others. To have a clean heart you must always get rid of bad thoughts and keep your judgments and intentions good. When you are curious about everyone's business, it is a sign that your heart needs some clean up. Knowing everyone else's business can fuel your imagination. Purity means filling your own mind with thoughts of Jesus. Instead of being curious about other people's personal business, spend time contemplating what it means being a daughter of the King. These sorts of thoughts lead to a pure heart for Christ.

Here are some possible goals to help you to have a pure heart:

- Dress in clothing befitting of your dignity of a Daughter of the King
- Wear appropriate clothing for the occasion
- Cultivate your inner beauty by avoiding TV shows and movies that attack human dignity and modesty
- Read magazines that refrain from vulgar photos and stories; Remember, you will be treated as you act and dress
- Keep your mind focused on your own stuff and stay out of other people's business
- Always assume the best about people
- Always give people the benefit of the doubt until you know the "facts"
- Go to confession if you need to detox your heart.
- Read about girl saints to stay focused on purity of heart, mind and body

Maria Goretti had a pure heart and mind. She valued this gift and was willing to die for her purity. You may not have to die for this virtue, but you will have to work for it in today's world. Pray and ask Maria to help you. You will be glad you asked!

Examination of Conscience

Do I give everyone, even those I don't like, the benefit of the doubt?

Do listen to music with vulgar words or impure messages?

Do I watch television shows or movies that have impure actions?

Do I think revengeful thoughts when someone does something unkind to me?

Do I wear clothing that may cause others to have impure thoughts?

Am I curious about other's bodies?

Am I careful to keep my private parts to myself?

Do I try to only say nice things about people?

Am I curious about other people's business?

Do I eavesdrop on other people's conversations?

History of Fashion

In the late 1890's and early 1900's women were very respected. However, there were not a lot of opportunities as far as careers. Motherhood and homemaking were esteemed. The clothing reflected these attitudes. Dresses and skirts were long, past the ankle, high necklines, and puffy sleeves. The undergarments were very restricting.

The corset was what every woman wore in those days. A corset is a miserable undergarment that was laced in the back and the laces were pulled extremely tight to make the waist tiny. Women were not very mobile to say the least. Hair was worn very long and loosely knotted at the top of the head. This style was quite elaborate. Hats were all the rage and were also elaborate and brims were very wide.

Then came the roaring twenties! Women cut their hair into the popular bob style and ditched the corset in favor of a loose camisole. The look was to have the figure of a boy. Women still didn't have the opportunities we have today but more women were educated and held jobs such as secretaries, teachers and nurses. For the first time women went to bars, drank, and smoked for recreation. Slowly, women were becoming less restricted.

Here are some of the popular styles during this era:

- Skirts above the ankle.
- Dropped waistlines that gave the "boy" body shape.
- Long beads.
- Strappy pointed toe shoes.

The nineteen thirties marked a time when the economy took a dive. Many people lost their wealth, homes, jobs or farms. Life once again became more serious. The clothing reflected this. More practical and tailored attire was popular.

- Skirts were still above the ankle, but the "boy" silhouette was replaced with a more feminine figure
- For undergarments women wore bras
- Blouses, jackets, and simple dresses were the norm
- For the celebs, fur was very popular with it embellishing coats and used for muffs and hats; If you were super rich you would wear a fur coat
- Traditional pumps

The nineteen forties brought World War II, which took America out of the depression of the thirties. Men left their families to fight over seas. For the first time women took over the jobs of men. They worked in factories that built the airplanes. They headed up volunteer organizations. Everyone's efforts went to helping the boys fighting. The clothing showed the somber atmosphere of the country and the lack of materials.

- Knee length hemlines
- Women, for the first time, wore pants to work, but skirts or dresses were worn out in public
- Tailored tops and jackets with large shoulder pads symbolizing the responsibilities women were undertaking.
- A-line skirts
- Platform shoes and pumps with rounded toe
- Pleated trousers, resembling men's attire

The nineteen fifties brought a time of prosperity. The war was over and people began to open businesses, buy cars and women had the luxury of once again being homemakers. By this time though, many more women were able to support themselves because of higher education. After the war, it was as if women hard proven their abilities. However, women embraced their femininity through their clothing.

- A defined waist and very fitted bodice and full skirts accentuated the feminine figure
- Knee length and long full skirts were popular
- All clothing was very fitted
- Capri pants became popular and were called pedal pushers
- Rolled up jeans and penny loafers were worn by teenagers
- Girdles and bras were essential for women to achieve the feminine figure for the clothing

The nineteen sixties began a revolution we can still see going on today. Women and men began to throw away the morals of their parents. Young people questioned purity and marriage opting to "experiment" with traditional beliefs and practices. This entire attitude showed in the fashions of the day.

- Hemlines rose to above the knee and the mini skirt was born
- Halter-tops and short shorts became popular
- Many women had bra-burning parties
- The hippy look was born
- Jackie Kennedy was the icon of true fashion of the era wearing pillbox hats and boxy suit jackets; She is still considered a fashion idol today

The nineteen seventies took what the sixties started and expanded on it. Women's "lib" started and the feminist movement was defined. See Girls Rock! for a detailed explanation on feminism and it's ideas. Here are some of the things that were popular for the seventies.

- Styles from the 40's reappeared such as platform shoes and A lined skirts
- Ponchos and "maxi" skirts appeared as did jumpsuits
- Hip huggers and bell-bottoms were all the rage
- Body suits and cropped tops were popular with teens
- Halter-tops

In the 80's many women went to college and had careers. There were many options in fashion that included a variety of skirt lengths and pants were popular. Other things that women wore were:

- Jackets, blouses and virtually all tops had large shoulder pads and oversized sweaters were a favorite
- Leggings, pleated pants and straight leg jeans
- Argyle sweaters and vests
- Polo shirts, oxford button down blouses
- Wide belts and pointed toe pumps

The nineteen nineties went back to more conservative styles. The first Iraq war influenced the fashions during this era. Women wore:

- Short skirt lengths
- Fitted tops and jackets with no shoulder pads
- Wide legged pants; Low rise slacks and jeans
- Chunky healed shoes

What do you think will be the fashions of the future? Look back over the decades to make your predictions. Remember, nothing is ever really new, it's just recycled. If you keep things long enough, say 30 years you can resurrect them!

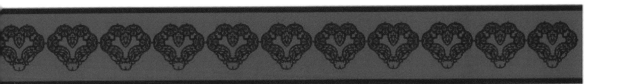

Can we Talk about Girl Talk?

Ladies, and I do mean 'Ladies,' the virtues of purity and modesty go beyond your appearance. They also move into the realm of how you act and speak. There's nothing worse than a nice girl that has a potty mouth. And guess what! Boys hate it, too. They see you as one of the 'guys' and not someone to respect and admire. As much as girls, and even women, think they are "liberated" and that they can look, act and talk like truck drivers, guys like girls to be ladies. This is especially true when it comes to toilet talk. One day I made a comment to my teenage son about a girl in his class who I thought was nice. To my surprise he said he didn't like her. When I asked why, he said it was because she used bad language. Girls, you are a daughter of the King! It is not fitting your status to have a trashy mouth! Girls who use bad language find that it becomes a hard to break habit…so don't go down that path.

What exactly does this mean? Well, here are a few pointers for you, a princess in the royal family of God:

- *If you can't say something nice, don't say anything at all*
- *Vulgar language is NOT an option*
- *Swearing is a NO-NO*
- *Dirty jokes are to be avoided. If someone tells one around you either walk away or say something like, " Real nice…," "That's disgusting!" or "Keep it to yourself next time."*
- *Name-calling is not nice, so don't do it*
- *Conversation about personal bodily functions is tacky, so skip it*
- *Talking about personal "girl" stuff should be done privately with mom*

As a rule of thumb, if you couldn't say it in front of our Blessed Mother, don't say it. Remember, she's in Heaven and would hear you anyway! One day all will have to give an accounting, before God, of every word that has been said. That should cause some serious hesitation before speaking! Imagine, every word matters. Did you know that long ago God told Abraham that everyone who cursed Abraham would be cursed and that everyone who blessed Abraham would be blessed? God was saying, "I listen to everything everyone says."

Whatever comes out of the mouth is there forever. It can't be taken back. The tongue can be as sharp as a two edged sword. Don't use it as a weapon and don't use it to lower your dignity as a princess so toss the toilet talk! You'll be glad you did.

Here's a very old story to help you remember the power of words:

Many hundreds of years ago, in a Jewish village, was a man who had spoken quite poorly to his neighbor and then, as time went by, even more viciously about this neighbor to others. One day this man began to feel regret over his unkind words and went to see his rabbi. He walked all day to the synagogue and all the while his regret grew. Finally, he arrived at the temple and found the Rabbi.

"Rabbouni, I have made a terrible mistake. I have spoken terribly to my neighbor and made things worse by saying bad things about my neighbor's character to others. What should I do?"

The rabbi thought for a while and then said, "You have to go back to your home and take your bed pillow and walk to the edge of our village where I want you to open up the pillow and shake the feathers out into the wind. When you have done this, please come back to see me."

Well, the man did not understand why the rabbi made this odd request but did just as he was told. It took him all night to walk back to his home and get his pillow. It took him many more hours to walk to the edge of the village and open his pillow up and shake the feathers from inside of it out into the wind. The wind quickly lapped up the feathers and spread them farther than the eye could see. Once he was satisfied that he had done what the rabbi had asked, the man returned to the synagogue.

Exhausted, but pleased that he had followed the rabbi's instructions perfectly, the man said, "Rabbouni, I have done what you asked. I have spent many hours walking from one place to another and have released all the feathers of my pillow out into the winds. They have been taken far and wide."

"Perfect," the rabbi responded. "Now go gather the feathers back."

To which the man gasped. "Gather them back!?! Why, that is impossible to do. How can you ask such a thing?"

Revealing great wisdom and understanding the rabbi replied, "And so it is with your words. Once uttered, they are impossible to retrieve. They are scattered far and wide"

MAKEUP

SHOULD I OR SHOULDN'T I?

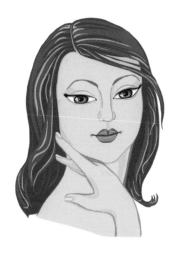

Your mother will give you the final answer to that question. Remember: whatever she says, goes! When she does say that you are able to start wearing makeup, there is something you must keep in mind.

Always show that you are a daughter of the King. Like your clothes, words, and behavior; makeup should be modest as well. But what does that mean? Simply, it means that you shouldn't look like you have makeup on. It should enhance your natural beauty, maybe cover a blemish outbreak, and always protect you from harmful UV rays; but makeup shouldn't be obvious or overdone!

Here are a few tips when mom says it is okay for you to begin wearing makeup:

STEP 1: CONCEALER Use to cover blemishes, dark circles or other flaws; Choose a shade at least two shades lighter than your skin; Use a sponge applicator and dab on skin; Do not pull or tug the skin

STEP 2: FOUNDATION Choose a foundation EXACTLY your skin color; Use a foundation with at least SPF 15; Choose foundation to go with your skin type (ex: oil free, cream to powder or liquid); Use a sponge applicator and dab makeup in spots all over face and eye lids; Blend in gently in an outward motion; Don't apply under the chin or on the neck

STEP 3: POWDER Use a large natural hair brush to apply loose or pressed powder; Tap brush on the edge of the container to knock off the excess; Apply in a downward motion

STEP 4: EYE MAKEUP There are many techniques to use with different eye shapes. The following application works for all shapes; Use natural hair eye shadow brush; Knock excess powder; Apply lightest shadow from brow to lashes; Select a darker shade in the same color family and apply to the crease and eyelid; Use a darker brown, charcoal or black to line the upper lash line only; If you line lower, it will close in the eye; Apply mascara from bottom of lashes to the top. Do not "pump" the tube; Discard mascara tube after 6-12 weeks to avoid eye infections

STEP 5: EYEBROW ARCH Follow the natural arch of the brow; Fill in the brow with a natural brown eye shadow that matches; Shadow is softer than a pencil; The end of the brow should end at the corner of the eye; As a side note, tweeze or wax stray brows for a clean, finished look. Do not make them too thin; Stay with the natural arch.

STEP 6: BLUSH Blush is applied to give contour to the face, not for "rosy cheeks"; Use a natural hair brush if using a powder and knock off excess; If using a cream or liquid, use your fingers or a sponge, apply a couple dots and blend from end of nose at the outside corner of the eye, underneath the cheek bone, near the hair line, toward the ear; Apply powder the same way

STEP 7: LIPSTICK AND LIP LINER Always use a lip liner; Use short, feathery strokes to outline the lips; Choose a liner in the same color family as the lipstick; Fill in with lip liner and go over with lipstick; Using lip brush will make your application cleaner; Add gloss

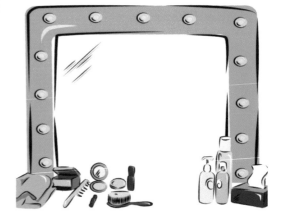

What's in My Closet?

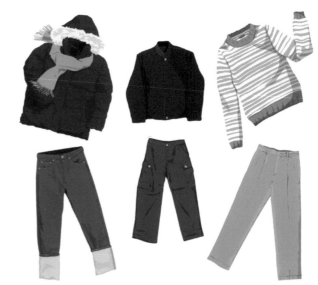

○ Do I have anything in my wardrobe that would offend Our Lord? If so, what?

○ Do I need to get rid of any piece/s of clothing that are not modest? If so, what?

○ What would Jesus say to me about the way I dress for school, out with friends, Church, to formals?

○ Do I have a submissive or rebellious spirit concerning dress?

○ Modesty protects the intimate center of the person. Do I show my commitment to keeping this intimate center veiled?

○ Do I take care to dress properly so that I do not cause another to sin in mind or deed?

○ Do I realize I am the daughter of the King and dress and act accordingly?

○ Jesus dwells in the tabernacle of every Catholic Church. When I attend mass do I dress in my best clothes to give God honor and glory? If no, why?

○ Do I take care that my swimsuit does not reveal what should remain hidden and keep a beach cover-up close so that I may cover myself when out of the water?

First Impressions

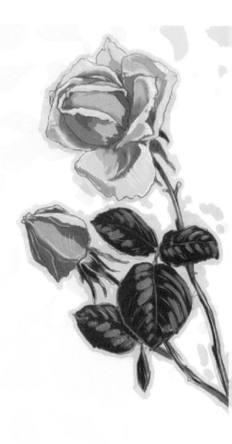

How you act, dress, and speak says something about who you are as a person. Yes it's true; we all make judgments on first impressions. No, it's not right to judge people, but we all do it even if it is quite unconsciously. Making a bad impression can cause you to lose a friendship, embarrass your parents, or when you're older it can cause you to lose a job opportunity. It only takes thirty seconds to make an impression and it's difficult to get a second chance. Here are a few things you can do to make a good impression:

- Wear clothing appropriate for the occasion.
- Always appear clean and neat.
- Don't try to look older than you are.
- Be polite when being introduced to someone new.
- Look the person in the eye.
- Smile.

Things like wearing too much makeup or dressing immodestly are two good ways to ruin a first impression. As a daughter of the King, you will want to live up to your royal status and always make a good impression.

You've Gotta Have a Plan!

You know it is important to take care of and control your body. In the same way, you need to take care of your soul. You need to nourish it so that it can grow in friendship with Jesus. How is that done? You gotta have a plan!

Do you think athletes make it to the Olympics by chance? Do you think they go with the flow and train here and there and somehow one day they end up in the Olympic games winning a medal? Of course not, you know that! They have a plan that includes diet and training. They follow it everyday, even when they don't feel like it. This dedication allows the athlete to attain their goal, their dream of winning a medal at the Olympics.

Think about the purpose of your life, to know, love and serve God in this life and to be happy with Him forever in the next. Do you think you can achieve this goal without some planning and preparation?

Here's a simple but effective plan you can use your entire life to complete your training here and attain your Heavenly goal. You can also use the special "All Things Girl" journal to write your own plan, prayers, and thoughts.

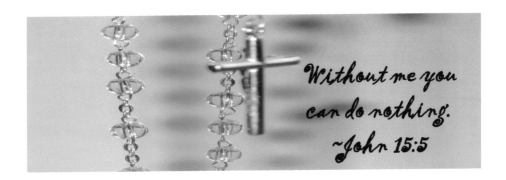

Without me you can do nothing.
~John 15:5

WHAT THINGS SHOULD BE PART OF YOUR PLAN?

MORNING OFFERING:

A good way to start your day is to say, "Hello, Jesus!" The day ahead is a great gift from God. The morning offering consists of giving Jesus everything you will do and say that day. Tell Him you want to please Him and give Him glory in all that you do.

You can make up your own special prayer or you can choose one to memorize. For example, here's a very simple prayer.

"Good Morning dear Jesus this day is for you, I ask you to bless all that I say and do. Amen"

Or ... *"Oh Jesus through the Immaculate Heart of Mary I offer you the prayers, works, joys, and sufferings of this day, For all the intentions of Your Sacred Heart, in union with the Holy Sacrifice of the Mass said throughout the world today, in reparation for my sins, for the intentions of all our associates, and for the intentions of the Holy Father this month. Amen"*

It is important to try and say your morning offering at the same time every day so that you remember to do it. Some girls will say it right when they wake up. Others, when they sit down to breakfast. Whatever works for you, just do it!

DAILY PRAYER.

Prayer is talking to Jesus. It is something great! Jesus prayed and openly encouraged his disciples to pray. And guess what? You, as a daughter of the King, are a disciple. How does a person learn to pray? Start out by setting aside 5 minutes of your day to sit down in a quiet place where there will be no distractions. Place yourself in the presence of Jesus, asking your guardian angel to help you start a conversation with Jesus. Because prayer is an intimate conversation with God, you can talk to God as your best friend and tell Him the things that are concerning you, what is making you happy, angry or sad; God is always listening. You may tell Him something like: *"Hi Jesus, guess what I'm doing today? I'm going to my cousins' house! Mom said I have to clean my room before going....and you know Jesus, I hate cleaning my room! But I guess I'll do it.... Maybe I should offer it up for a special intention, eh? Who needs prayers, Jesus?....."* On you go. You are praying! Slowly increase the 5 minutes of prayer a day to 10 minutes. You will feel so happy when you spend time talking to Jesus every day!

THE ROSARY OF THE BLESSED MOTHER. Do you enjoy looking at family pictures and remembering those precious moments? Well, when you pray the rosary you contemplate moments in the lives of Jesus and Mary on each mystery. The rosary is divided into 4 parts: each part into five mysteries. For each mystery one Our Father and Ten Hail Mary's are prayed while you meditate on a certain time of Jesus' life. The name rosary means "crown of roses". Think about each of the Hail Mary's you pray as a rose offered to Our Lady. By the end of the rosary, you have offered her a huge bouquet of beautiful roses! If saying the entire rosary seems like a big task, start out with just one decade and slowly add one at a time. The idea is to make the effort and to keep on trying.

EXAMINATION OF CONSCIENCE AT NIGHT. Before going to bed, it's a good idea to take a quick look at your day in God's presence to see if you have behaved as a daughter of the King. An easy way to do this is by asking yourself these three questions:

- *What did I do today that was pleasing to God?*
- *What did I do today that was not pleasing to God?*
- *What does God want me to do better tomorrow?*

Ponder briefly on each question, and then follow with an act of contrition to tell Jesus that you are sorry for having offended Him. An Act of Contrition is just a short prayer telling Jesus you are sorry for your sins. It can be as simple as *"I'm sorry, Lord. Help me do better tomorrow."* Or it can be the traditional Act of Contrition, *" Oh my God, I am heartily sorry for having offended thee and I detest all my sins because of the loss of Heaven and the pains of Hell, But most of all because they offend Thee my God who are all good and deserving of all my love. I firmly resolve with the help of Thy grace, to confess my sins, to do penance and to amend my life, Amen."*

PRAY THREE HAIL MARY'S AT NIGHT BEFORE GOING TO BED ASKING THE BLESSED MOTHER TO HELP YOU KEEP YOUR HEART PURE.

Don't delay, start today, you can win the Olympics of the spiritual life!

A GIRL LIKE ME!

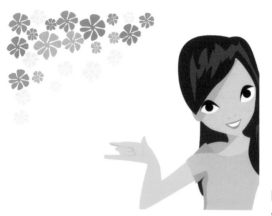

The Story of St. Maria Goretti

Maria Goretti is a saint for the modern world. She is an excellent example of a young girl who valued her dignity as a daughter of God. Maria was born on October 16, 1890 in a town called Corinaldo, Italy. Her parents were hardworking, but poor. Her father died when she was ten and her mother worried about how to make ends meet. Mrs. Goretti had to move in with a family named Serenelli.

In this family was the father, John, and a son, Alessandro. Alessandro was about 20 years old and had very vile habits such as drinking and looking at pornographic magazines. It was a difficult time for Mrs. Goretti but she did her best for her family. Maria, too, did her best. She would say to her mother, "Be brave, Mother. After all, we're growing up. Soon we'll all be able to work and support the whole family and until then, God will provide for us." She helped her mother care for her younger brothers and sisters with jobs around the home.

During this time, Maria's mother worked outside of the home. Maria was left to tend the children. Over and over again, during the day, Alessandro would pester Maria to do impure things with him. Maria adamantly refused and told him such things were sins. She became very frightened to stay home alone. It was a terrible time for Maria as she wanted to make things easier for her mother but also had to contend with the terrible ways in which Alessandro treated her.

One day, while everyone was outside thrashing beans, Alessandro came back to the house where he grabbed a long piece of sharpened iron. He called to Maria. She froze. He seized her as she struggled, saying, "No, God doesn't want it, it is a sin." She fought until he took the sharp piece of iron and furiously stabbed her. After the attack, Alessandro, thinking her dead, turned and went into his room. Maria lay bleeding and in extreme pain. She dragged herself to the door and called for help. As Alessandro heard her, he came out of the room and stabbed her six more times then went into his room again and barred the door. Her mother and friends frantically tried to bandage Maria's wounds and took her to the hospital. Maria Goretti knew that her body was a temple to the Holy Spirit and sadly had to die to protect it.

At the hospital, a priest was called to hear Maria's confession and give her last rights. She was asked if she forgave her attacker and she replied, "I do forgive him and I believe that God will forgive him, too." Maria died in the hospital. She was not quite 12 years old but she knew how important her purity was to herself and to God. Maria died in 1902 and was canonized in 1950. Alessandro, who had experienced a conversion and repentance while in prison, was at the side of Maria's mother for the canonization.

As a young woman in today's world, it is hard to resist the thought that the body is the most important thing about you or that it has to look a certain way to be beautiful. The truth is: you are the "person" who you are because you are a daughter of the King. In Christ is where your true beauty lies.

St. Maria Goretti is an example of the true beauty of purity. You should know that you can always pray to St. Maria Goretti for the courage to be pure!

The fruits of the Spirit are perfections that the Holy Spirit forms in us as the first fruits of eternal glory. The tradition of the Church lists twelve of them: "Charity, joy, peace, patience, kindness, goodness, generosity, gentleness, faithfulness, modesty, self-control, chastity."

CCC# 1832

LaVergne, TN USA
15 September 2010
197132LV00001B